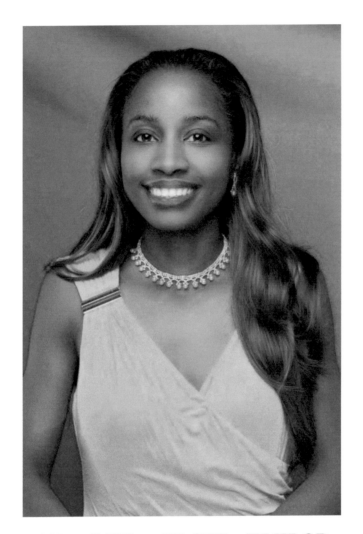

BY: REV. TASHA TAYLOR

"TABLE OF CONTENTS"

"INTRODUCTION"

In Philippians 4:13 the Bible says, "I can do all things through Christ who strengthens me." This was always one of my favorite scriptures. I think that this scripture is pronounced because it demands a level of faith that not every other believer may possess. This faith is the, "Gift of Faith." I encourage you to read on it. It will change your life. God Bless you.

CHAPTER 1.

"NOW FAITH: CONCERNING HEALING"

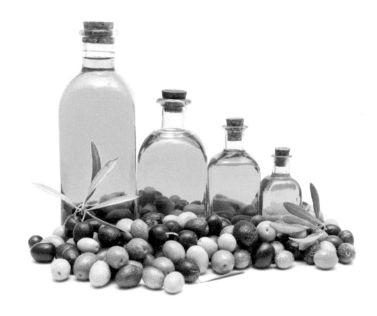

According to, Hebrews 11:1, "Now Faith is the substance of things hoped for, the evidence of things not seen." One might be concerned with how Faith connects with one's healing. Matter of fact, there is a time in the Bible where Jesus said, "Your Faith has made you whole." Matthew 9:22 says, "But Jesus turned Him about, and when He saw her, He said, 'Daughter, be of good comfort: thy Faith hath made thee whole: And the woman was made whole from that hour." Directly after this verse Jesus rose another woman from the dead. Faith activates Supernatural power into the atmosphere. This is why multiple healings can take place at the same time, because people's Faith are built up through seeing miracles. This sets the atmosphere for supernatural occurrences. On my Church prayer-line one person was healed of a foot issue after the testimony was given several others were also healed of foot or leg issues. It is not that the power of healing is limited in that area, but that people's Faith are increased concerning foot issues so the evidence keeps reoccurring in that area.

The power of Testimonials are so important, because it defeats the enemy, while increasing ones Faith. Also, it charges other people's Spirit Man and they are able to seek God for their healing. The Bible says in Isiah 53:5, "But He was wounded for our transgressions, He was bruised for our iniquities: the chastisement of our peace was upon Him; and with His stripes we are healed. " The Grace of Jesu brought Salvation and healing; inadvertently the same Faith it takes to receive Salvation is the same Faith one needs for healing. Healing is a gift of the Spirit that Jesus performed almost daily once He left the wilderness. His time of testing prepared Him for greatness. The Bible says in Matthew 15:26, "But He answered and said, it is not meet to take the children's bread and to cast it to dogs." Jesus is referring healing to bread to Gods' children. It is a necessity for Gods' children to receive healing. God is our Jehovah Rapha (Jer. 30:17; Jer. 3:22; Isa. 30:26; Isa. 61:1;

Psa. 103:3). Healing takes place in
deliverance, backslidings, diseases and
wounds. Healing in comparison to bread
shows how vital, often and how our very
lives depend on it. Without healing we would
be deprived the vital gift we need for
Spiritual survival. Once a believer is
saved his or hers health is attacked by the
enemy as an act of Spiritual warfare. Job
endured graciously. In order to defeat the
enemy we need daily healing in areas of our
lives that only God sees. Man believers are

wounded emotionally on a daily basis for living for Christ; without healing many people's hearts would fail.

In order to defeat the devil we need daily healing in areas of our lives that only God sees. Many believers might be wounded emotionally or on a daily basis while living for Christ; without healing many people's hearts would fail. It is important for believers to pray daily for healing in all areas so that they are not, "weary and heavy laden." The Bible says in Matthew 11:28-29,

"Come unto me, all that are

heavy laden, and I will give

you rest. Take my yoke upon

you and learn of me; for I am

meek and lowly in heart: and

ye shall find rest unto your

souls."

Often time's believers find themselves heavy
laden with the cares of this world,

tragedies, crisis, trials and tribulations. In order for believers to withstand the wiles of the enemy they must experience full healing; Thus exude the Joy of the Lord. "...The Joy of the Lord is our Strength" the

Bible says in, Nehemiah 8:10. When we show the fruit of Joy it shows that the fruit of healing has been manifested in our lives. Healing cause's believers to live lives free of hurt, shame and regret and liberates believers to have hope, which makes them not ashamed. The Holy Bible States:[i]

And hope maketh not ashamed;

Because the love of God is

shed abroad in our hearts by

the Holy Ghost which is given

unto us. For when we were yet

without strength, in due time

Christ died for the ungodly.

For scarcely for a righteous man

will one die: yet peradventure

for a good man some would even

dare to die. But God commendeth

his love toward us, in that, while

we were yet sinners, Christ died

for us. Much more then, being now

justified by his blood, we shall

be saved from wrath through him.

For if, when we were enemies, we

were reconciled to God by the death

of his Son, much more, being

reconciled, we shall be saved by his

life. And not only so, but we also

joy in God through our Lord Jesus

Christ, by whom we have now

received the atonement.

Hope is the very factor that helps the
heart to heal. The Bible says, "Hope
deferred maketh the heart sick: but when the
desire cometh, it is a tree of life" in
Proverbs 13:12. Hope helps the heart to
envision, dream and see fulfillment in

promises. God created mankind in His image.
God saw what He wanted, spoke it and the
Word became flesh and dwelt among us; also,
the worlds was formed by His Word and His
Word is not changing. God communed with
Himself and decided to make man in His own
image including the ability to see, envision

and dream. Without the ability to hope a
person is deemed hopeless because he or she
chooses not to see, envision or dream
anything for themselves. Therefore, they
are left to help fulfill the vision of

another or end up tragically not fulfilling their destiny. The very fact that God gave man a soul shows a connection with their Creator God. The Bible says that, "Then the LORD God formed a man from the dust of the ground and breathed into his nostrils the breath of life, and the man became a living being," in Genesis 2:7. The very breath in man should show some connection with His Creator. For a person to be deemed heartless it is to say the person lacks a soul, when undoubtedly God made everyone with a soul.

However, when someone denies and denounces the very existence of God, they begin to cut themselves away from their life source and become hopeless, vision less, fruitless and believes their life is a factor of chance instead of promise. This hopeless mindset leads people to homosexual behaviors and irreconcilable behavior like suicide and blasphemy. Hopelessness, is a fruit of faithlessness and once someone loses the Faith it is hard to win them back over. The Bible says that, once you have tasted of the light and then turn away it is harder to be won back (I paraphrase).[ii]

You might think why would one walk away from Faith, or, their belief in the sovereign God. Is it not evident in the American Culture today? Greed causes people to tread in places they ought not to be for more power, wealth ad influence. People are always seeking more. The Bible says, Godliness and contentment is great gain in I Timothy 6:6. However, as much as societies have advanced in history both the Godly and ungodly share a common factor, their lust for more. This lust or greed led them into paganism, separating them from God and leading to their demise. America has always only trusted in God, because our founding fathers allowed the Bible to be taught in schools. Today, Harry Potter's books have been used in Public School curriculum to teach our children. What a wide factor and margin to compare and contrast. Yesterday's children raised families with virtuous women with morals and standards in their households.

The lack of Faith in our society today has increased substitutes and cults that do not believe in structure, thus leaving our families without father figures in the home. God set structure of God first, the man and then the woman; but without God, leading a home or family structure in our society has had devastating results. In today's culture men and men, worst lesbians are free to raise families. The confusion has left our society bewildered, in a state of hopelessness; thus, leading to more crimes, high rates of suicide among adults and children because we fail to teach Faith, the Bible. According to Wikipedia, "Research has found that attempted suicide rates and suicidal ideation among lesbian, gay, bisexual, transgender, etc. (LGBT) youth is significantly higher than among the general population.[1] LGBT youth have the highest rate of suicide attempts."[iii]

CHAPTER 2:

"NOW FAITH: CONCERNING DELIVERANCE"

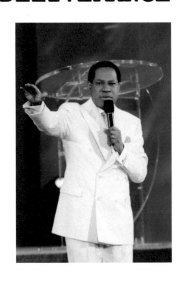

Deliverance is a long word, and as it is a long word, it is a long process. Jesus encouraged us believers to pray and fast, because some strong holds are not easily broken.[iv] When believers begin to fast and pray strongholds are broken and the person getting deliverance can be freed from unclean spirits. When one operates in Exousia Power[v] unclean spirits leave because they recognize the power and authority one walks in. When Jesus cast out the devil out of the dumb and mute man he immediately began speaking; because, God is All Powerful.[vi] Power is known and recognized by all other forces and powers. We know this because the Bible talks about spiritual wickedness in high places, these are forms and levels of powers, including the occult, demonic forces, etc… All these "powers" are subjected to the All Mighty and All Powerful God that we serve as believers in Christ Jesus. Once one believes that Jesus is Lord, he or she is submitting to the highest Power there is. The Bible says,

"Every knee shall bow and every tongue shall confess that Jesus Christ is Lord."[vii] The powers that be must subject themselves to the Almighty God; whether or not they choose to follow the occult all must bow to Jesus.

Deliverance is a choice. When one chooses to release the mindset of the occult and say yes to Jesus that Faith to do so will set them free. One must choose be delivered. In the Bible the man with the legion began screaming and begging Jesus, but the demons inside the man pled not to be cast out. However, the man did not want the burden of thousands of demons inside of him so he began to scream. So Jesus delivered the man from the thousands of devils inside him making it hopeful for that man to lead and live a normal life.

When one is possessed of the devil the spirit of hopelessness takes over, and despair. The individual no longer feels like living, because he chooses not to hope.

The Bible say, "hope makes not ashamed...," in Romans 5:5. A life without hope is one full of shame and despair. Many times people resort to drinking alcohol not understanding why. It is because they have lost hope and accepted that there is nothing they can di, even God to help their situation. Which is why God calls them fools because, "For with God nothing shall be impossible."[viii]

People who fail to hope, fail to believe and fail about everything there is

in life; because, they choose not to believe
God as their way of escape. This mindset
leads ones like this to depression, then
suicidal behaviors like drugs, marijuana,
depressants, and eventually suicide. One
might ask why our society is so filled with
suicidal deaths. It is because our society
is becoming faithless in the One True All
Powerful God. We must repent. One might
say who must repent? I conclude the
righteous and we must stand up and pray that
God restores the Faith, hope and the Spirit
of God in this nation. One might say show

me evidence of backsliding? We have left the cross and turned to mammon. The Holy Scriptures says, "We can't serve both God and mammon;" however, if you turn over your dollar bill someone in "power," thinks it's possible to do so. Pray that God restores the Faith of our nation.

CHAPTER 3:

"NOW FAITH: CONCRNING PROSPERITY"

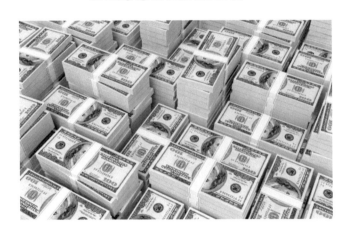

The Bible says, "Above all things I wish that you prosper as your soul prospers," in 3 John 1:2. Just as much as God wants our soul in Heaven, He wants us to physically, socially, emotionally, educationally… prosper. God wants you to prosper in every area of your life. It is not Gods will that you are destitute. The Bible says, "You have not because you ask not" in James 4:2. God wants us to ask Him for everything we need. It is not Biblical to be introverted because we must actively seek out what we

need from people as well. If 10 people say,
"no" the odds that the next 10 will also
say, "no" is highly impossible. Somebody is
going to help you if you seek out help. God
doesn't want you hungry, there are

agencies on every corner giving out free
food samples or pantry supplies. We have
not because we ask not is the reality of the
situation.

It's time to open up our mouths and seek
for help. In my book, "Success and its
Enemy Called Crisis" the theme is that

"Success Begins When Asking For Help." Stop waiting for people to read your mind and say "I Need Help!" People do not understand the term Fund Raiser anymore, because they might not have a desire to give; however, if they see the need because you are asking God work a miracle for you. Stop seeking a "psychic" which is a lesser "power" and activate Gods' Word which is the, Highest Power. In Matthew 7:7, "Ask and it will be given to you; seek and you will find; knock and

the door will be opened to you." These Biblical principles will lead one to success every time. Ask and it will be given to you; seek and you will find; knock and the door will be opened to you. It's not going to happen by works only, also use Faith. Move on it! Now!

What is God showing you now? What is God telling you now? What is God revealing to you now? Move on it! Where is God taking you now? What is God doing for you now? Be Thankful! Your miracle is activated when your Faith level moves with your expectancy now!

CHAPTER 4

"NOAHS' FAITH PRESERVING

HIS FAMILY"

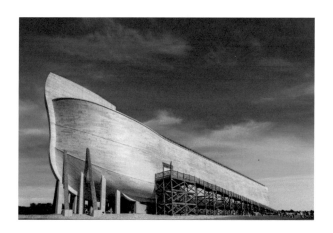

When God cast satan out of Heaven, he corrupted mankind with the fall, then the devils that left Heaven with him began mating with humans. Human beings began to look monstrous. When God cast satan out of Heaven, he corrupted mankind with the fall, then the devils that left Heaven with him began mating with humans. Human beings began to look monstrous, with superpowers, the Bible states, "...and they bare children to them, the same became mighty men which were of old, men of reknown."[ix] Noah was

given a warning from God of pending

destruction, because God was going to wipe

out mankind for good; because, of the evil

on the earth. The Bible says in Genesis

6:6-7,

"And it repented the Lord that

He had made man on the earth, it

grieved Him at His heart. And

the Lord said, I will destroy

man whom I have created from the

face of the earth; both man, and

beast, and the creeping thing and

the fowls of the air; for it

repenteth me that I have made

them."

Then the Bible states, "But Noah found grace

in the eyes of the Lord."[x] This is Gods'

sovereignty. Noah had favor in the eyes of

God and Noah's family brought God hope.

Maybe, God saw that his families' structure

was in agreement with God's perfect plan.

Noah had one wife, and his three sons had

one wife as well. God thought it best to allow Godliness to flourish in the land of the living. And he allowed Noah, a Godly man, to choose two of each creature to spare from destruction. God wanted to preserve purity and do away with wickedness, because the wickedness of the wicked was so great, they did not want to socialize or be around Noah and his family. They were the social outcast in this wicked community; which is why, when God shut the door only Noah and his family were inside and spared from distraction. Noah's Faith spared his household and his Faith was seen through the activation of Gods' will "now" or at that instant. As soon as God said it, Noah began to activate what God said to do, through his obedience at that instant. Noah did not wait for the rain to start or a flood to come before moving; neither, did he bother God with fleece. He immediately did what God told him to do.

CHAPTER 5:

"ISAIAH'S FAITH REBUILDING A TORN DOWN CITY, NATION, PEOPLE"

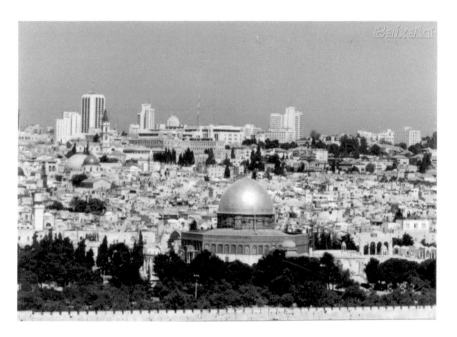

God desired a Holy people to Himself of the
Jewish community; however, they were lusting
for what the other nations had. They wanted
power, wealth and influence they did not
want God to lead them through the Prophets
anymore. This led to the Nations decline,
because, God gave them what they desired, a
new leader; and, one who would tell them
what to do. They were tired of waiting for
the prophets to deliver a message. They
wanted a quicker response from a king. A

king who would rule in their favor or lusts, and God gave them Saul.

King Saul was a rebel who wanted to do things his way. Gods' way was never enough, because Saul sought after the attention and favor of the people. He even showed the people that he could expedite. When he thought the Prophets fell short and lit the incense in the Temple because the Prophet took too long.[xi] This angered the Lord and the Spirit of God began leaving Saul. The people had no clue how angry this made God

and continued serving Saul and had Faith in
him. They began to trust in him not knowing
he was leading their Nation into demise.
Before they could get adjusted to their
crisis situation they were under attack and
Saul committed suicide and his sons were
killed by the Philistines sword. God had
gotten the victory and replaced Saul with
David. And the Nation was restored again.
However, the people put their trust in David
who killed Uria.[xii] He also committed

adultery and let sin corrupt his throne. Later, David was replaced by his son Solomon the last good king to the throne in the Old Testament. Then the Prophet Isiah warns Israel of their sins and all their backslidings hoping to restore them to God again. And the Prophet prophecies in Isaiah 61 that God will rebuild the desolations of many Generations. Isaiah prophecies of the hope to come through Jesus the Messiah.

The next time Jesus returns He will rapture the Church. Then the "Battle of Armageddon will take place and there will be war. The Bible says that the brightness of His appearing will slay the nations in II The. 2:8.The Bible says, "Every knee shall bow and every tongue shall confess that Jesus Christ is Lord."xiii

God promised through the Prophet Isaiah that they will have, "…beauty for ashes, the oil of joy for mourning and the garment of praise for the Spirit of heaviness."xiv Also, that we shall be kings and priest as God judges the earth that we will be there ruling with God too in that day when God divides the tears from the wheat, the sheep

from the goat and the sinners from the

righteous."[xv]

CHAPTER 6:

JESUS FAITH TO REACH THE NATIONS, REDEMPTION, SALVATION, AND HEALING

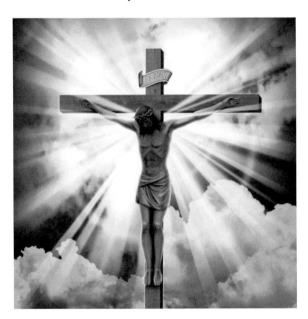

Jesus said, "He came unto His own, and His own received Him not. But as many as received Him, to them gave He power to become the sons of God, even to them that believe on His name:…"[xvi] True entitlement and son ship through Jesus Christ, comes through the Redemptive work on Calvary. When Jesus died on the cross, He rose up on the third day and reconciled us back to God. Due to the act of Salvation we who were once slaved to sin are reconciled to God through the act of the shedding of Blood on Calvary.

The Bible says, "And almost all things are by the law purged with blood; and without shedding of blood is no remission," in Hebrews 9:22. Sin is so costly, because it will cost one their life. We are only justified to God by Faith. The Bible says, "… but the just shall live by His faith."[xvii] Faith is the only thought process or belief that saves a man from condemnation. The Bible says, "Whoever believes in him is not condemned, but whoever does not believe stands condemned already because they have not believed in the name of God's one and only Son," in John 3:18. Our freedom of hope in Christ Jesus is to believe that, "Jesus died on the cross and believe in their heart that God rose Jesus up on the third day and confess with the ones mouth that Jesus is Lord![xviii] Salvation, Justification and the redemptive work on Calvary was done so that Jesus can save others by His Grace shown on the cross. If someone refuses the Grace of Jesus then they are a hopeless case. It would have been better for that person to not have been born. I think an untimely death would have been better one who died without Christ just to spare them the jeopardy of God's judgement to sinful man. "Jesus is the Way, the Truth and the Life and nobody goes to the Father but by Him." The Bible says, "Should we continue in sin because Grace abound," the writer Paul said, "God forbid."[xix] It is Gods will that we are free.

The Bible says, "He who the Son has set free is free indeed," in John 8:36.

Jesus died on the cross so that all souls, everywhere would be able to be reconciled to God the Father through the shedding of His Blood. The Blood of Jesus has All Power to break all chains and yokes, which is why every believer is set free from sin automatically when they confess their sin and receive the Blood of Jesus. Through the Blood of Jesus mankind is redeemed from sin and protected from the works of the devil.

As earlier said in this paper, God protects us from pestilence, sicknesses and diseases through the shedding of the Blood of Jesus on the cross of Cavalry. Mankind are redeemed, and justified by the finished work of Jesus on the cross and forgiven of all sin; because, Jesus rose Victoriously from the dead. Jesus did it all on the cross and defeated the devil, went down into hell and took the keys from satan; thus, giving us the Power to bind and loose. The Bible says, "Truly I tell you, whatever you bind on earth will be bound in heaven, and whatever you loose on earth will be loosed in Heaven," in Matthew 18:18.

We are given total victory, freedom and redemption when we confess in Faith that we believe in our heart that, "Jesus died on the cross and confess with our mouth that God raised Jesus from the dead and that Jesus is Lord."[xx]

CHAPTER 7:

"PAULS FAITH TO PICK UP THE MANTLE AND SPREAD THE GOOD NEWS TO JEWS AND GENTILES"

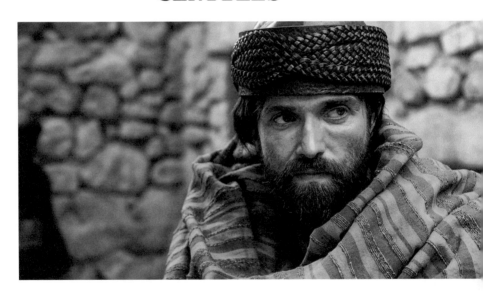

Paul was a Roman, because of this he was favored in his society. This may be why he outlived many of the disciples and brutally murdered as many of the disciples were. Instead, Paul was sentenced to banishment on the, "Isle of Patmos" by himself. Paul did not do as the others did, but he insisted to continue come what may. He had a divine visitation of the Lord and that changed his perception on what he had to do. Whether he had a boat or not, he made it to his destinations and delivered the message of Jesus being the Messiah and the Resurrection of Jesus. Paul never doubted as we see Peter did or lost hope and hid as the disciples after Jesus was crucified (but came out of hiding when He was risen) but Paul had purpose and motivation form within that could not be shaken. His Faith was on the solid rock. It was not movable. Whether he had a change of clothes to wear, or, not he was about the Fathers business and wrote 13 books in the Bible. Paul was a soul winner, a motivation and he was not moved by faces, but by the momentum of the, "Power of God" that was at work within him. Even in prison Paul sang songs of, "Praise and Worship" unto the Lord. His Faith was so strong that God sent Angels to rescue him repeatedly from prision.   His only accusation to his society was that he kept preaching in the name of Jesus; and, until he died, he continued to do just that. Nothing could move Paul, because he had a Rhema Word that was that, "Jesus was and is the Son of God slain from the foundations of the World."

CHAPTER 8:

"THE VIRTUOUS WOMAN"

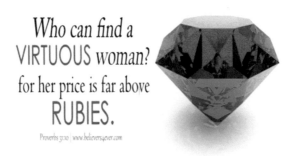

Who can find a VIRTUOUS woman? for her price is far above RUBIES.

Proverbs 31:10 | www.believers4ever.com

In the Holy Scriptures, the Bible talks about one of the Wisest, women noted, "The Virtuous Woman." The Bible says:

"Who can find a virtuous woman?

for her price is far above rubies.

The heart of her husband doth

safely trust in her, so that he

shall have no need of spoil. She

will do him good and not evil all

the days of her life. She

seeketh wool, and flax, and

worketh willingly with her hands.

She is like the merchants' ships;

She bringeth her food from afar.

She riseth also while it is yet

night, and giveth meat to her

household, and a portion to her

maidens. She considereth a field,

and buyeth it: with the fruit of

her hands she planteth a vineyard.

She girdeth her loins with strength,

and strengtheneth her arms. She

perceiveth that her merchandise

is good: her candle goeth not out

by night. She layeth her hands

to the spindle, and her hands

hold the distaff. She stretcheth

out her hand to the poor; yea, she

reacheth forth her hands to the

needy. She is not afraid of the

snow for her household: for all

her household are clothed with

scarlet. She maketh herself

coverings of tapestry; her

clothing is silk and purple. Her

husband is known in the gates,

when he sitteth among the elders

of the land. She maketh fine

linen, and selleth it; and

delivereth girdles unto the

merchant. Strength and honour

are her clothing; and she shall

rejoice in time to come. She

openeth her mouth with and in

her tongue is the law of

kindness. She looketh well to

the ways of her household, and

eateth not the bread of idleness.

Her children arise up, and call

her blessed; her husband also, and

he praiseth her. Many daughters

have done virtuously, but thou

excellest them all. Favour is

deceitful, and beauty is vain:

but a woman that feareth the Lord,

she shall be praised. Give her of

the fruit of her hands; and let

her own works praise her in the

gates."[xxi]

The virtuous woman has Faith that her preparation precedes her blessings. Therefore, her family is not hungry, is not cold, and is not disrespected and strong.

Her diligence to prepare causes her family

to praise her and celebrate her; because of

the mere fact that she inspires both men and

women to be more like her.

CHAPTER 9:

"THE QUEEN OF SHEEBA"

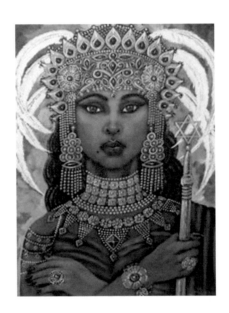

The excellence of this women is known generation from generation, because of her ability to detect greatness. She too was a woman of great wealth and influence, but her desire to leave a far distance to seek out Solomon a man of great wisdom, exposed that she was one too. Even though she was a woman, she attained wealth, favor and wisdom more that many men of her time. She was Queen and prospered so much because of her wisdom. She was one of a few in history to stand out as an extremely wealthy and prominent women. The Queen of Sheba, had

Faith that if she met Solomon he would

dazzle her and answer all her questions and

he did. The Bible records in I Kings 10:

When the queen of Sheba heard

about the fame of Solomon and

his relationship to the Lord,

she came to test Solomon with

hard questions. Arriving at

Jerusalem with a very great

caravan—with camels carrying

spices, large quantities

of gold, and precious

stones—she came to

Solomon and talked with him about

all that she had on her mind. 3

Solomon answered all her questions;

nothing was too hard for the king

to explain to her. When the queen

of Sheba saw all the wisdom of

Solomon and the palace he had built,

the food on his table, the seating

of his officials, the attending

servants in their robes, his

cupbearers, and the burnt

offerings he made at[a] the

temple of the Lord, she was

overwhelmed. She said to the

king, "The report I heard in my

own country about your

achievements and your wisdom is

true. But I did not believe

these things until I came and

saw with my own eyes. Indeed,

not even half was told me; in

wisdom and wealth you have

far exceeded the   report I

heard. How happy your people

must be! How happy your

officials, who continually

stand before you and hear

your wisdom! Praise be to

the Lord your God, who has

delighted in you and placed

you on the throne of Israel.

Because of the Lord's eternal

love for Israel, he has made

you king to maintain justice

and righteousness." And she

gave the king 120 talents[b]

of gold, large quantities

of spices, and precious

stones. Never again were so

many spices brought in as

those the queen of Sheba

gave to King Solomon. (Hiram's

ships brought gold from Ophir;

and from there they brought

great cargoes of almugwood[c]

and precious stones. The king

used the almugwood to make

supports[d] for the temple of

the Lord and for the royal

palace, and to make harps

and lyres for the musicians.

So much almugwood has never

been imported or seen since

that day.) King Solomon gave

the queen of Sheba all she

desired and asked for,

besides what he had given

her out of his royal bounty.

Then she left and returned
with her retinue to her own
country.

Sheba left the king even wealthier than
before because Solomon gave her riches from
his bounty. It is important to give gifts
to those in kingly positions because one can
gain favor and in this case, Sheba gained
more wealth. Her desire to bless the king
left her richer than before. In addition,
her reverence and Faith in his wisdom
allowed her to receive the answers she

desired.   Her Faith got her more wealth and

more wisdom.

CHAPTER 10:

"DEBORAH"

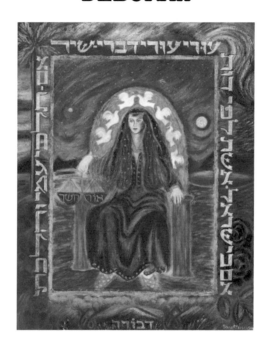

In the Bible that when Israel was given into slavery for 20 years that a woman named Deborah rose up to help to deliver Gods' people out of captivity. The Bible records:

"Certainly I will go with

you," said Deborah. "But

because of the course you

are taking, the honor will

not be yours, for the Lord

will deliver Sisera into the

hands of a woman." So

Deborah went with Barak to
Kedesh. 10 There Barak
summoned Zebulun and
Naphtali, and ten thousand
men went up under his command.
Deborah also went up with him.
Now Heber the Kenite had left
the other Kenites, the
descendants of Hobab, Moses'
brother-in-law,[b] and pitched

his tent by the great tree in

Zaanannim near Kedesh. When

they told Sisera that Barak son

of Abinoam had gone up to Mount

Tabor, 13 Sisera summoned from

Harosheth Haggoyim to the

Kishon River all his men and

his nine hundred chariots

fitted with iron. Then Deborah

said to Barak, "Go! This is

the day the Lord has given

Sisera into your hands. Has not

the Lord gone ahead of you?" So

Barak went down Mount Tabor,

with ten thousand men following

him. 15 At Barak's advance, the

Lord routed Sisera and all his

chariots and army by the sword,

and Sisera got down from his

chariot and fled on foot. Barak

pursued the chariots and army

as far as Harosheth Haggoyim,

and all Sisera's troops fell

by the sword; not a man was

left. 17 Sisera, meanwhile,

fled on foot to the tent of

Jael, the wife of Heber the

Kenite, because there was an

alliance between Jabin king

of Hazor and the family of

Heber the Kenite. Jael went
out to meet Sisera and said
to him, "Come, my lord, come
right in. Don't be afraid."
So he entered her tent, and she
covered him with a blanket.
"I'm thirsty," he said. "Please
give me some water." She opened
a skin of milk, gave him a
drink, and covered him up.

"Stand in the doorway of the tent," he told her. "If someone comes by and asks you, 'Is anyone in there?' say 'No.'" But Jael, Heber's wife, picked up a tent peg and a hammer and went quietly to him while he lay fast asleep, exhausted. She drove the peg through his temple into the ground, and he died. Just then Barak came by in pursuit of

Sisera, and Jael went out to meet

him. "Come," she said, "I will

show you the man you're looking

for." So he went in with her, and

there lay Sisera with the tent

peg through his temple—dead. On

that day God subdued Jabin king

of Canaan before the Israelites.

24 And the hand of the

Israelites pressed harder and

harder against Jabin king of

Canaan until they destroyed him.[xxii]

Deborah was a General in her own right and
had Faith that if she led the men in battle
that they would win. Indeed as she acted
upon her Faith instantaneously, the men won
the Battle. God is in Control!

"CONCLUSION"

What is God telling you now? What is God speaking to you now? Operate in Faith and get those things accomplished that God is leading you to do. If you could not do it God would not have asked you to do it.

Try God and watch your miracle unfold through Faith today.

"Biography"

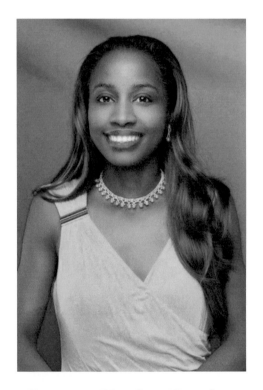

Pastor Tasha Taylor

Tasha Taylor was born in South Florida on September 21, 1982, to her parents Anthony Taylor and Sandra Mitchell. She was a gifted and talented songwriter from the age of 8 and sung in the children's choir at, Bethel First Assembly of God. There she was also baptized by Rev. James Peirce at the age of 12 and was filled with the Spirit with the evidence of speaking with other tongues as well. She wrote over 30 songs by the age of 15 and over 50 by the age of 18. Throughout Tasha's life she learned to pray and wait on God to be her vindicator, deliver and way maker. Through Tasha's

music God was able to make a way of
provision for Tasha during various financial

trials in her life. While attending,
"DayStar Ministries" Tasha was ordained an
"Evangelist" and served for over 20 years in
ministry.

Evangelist Tasha Taylor later attended
the "School of Prophets" in Miami, FL at the
"Rose of Sharon School of Biblical Studies"
and attended the "International Seminary"
satellite classes held there. Her first
year teacher was, Apostle Dr. Elizabeth

Hairston that has sowed a lot of prophecy in her life. Her second year teacher was none other than her mother, who also help found DayStar Ministries, Pastor Sandra Mitchell. Evangelist Tasha Taylor then attained her Bachelor's Degree from the International Seminary on February 2013. She began Pastoring her own church, "Reaping Time Outreach Global" at the age of 25. She was also newly married to her now ex-husband Michelet Josma. Their marriage lasted 7 years and they had a son named Joshua Josma.

Pastor Tasha Taylor began a Christian homeschool in her home and attempted to license 2 daycares in which 1 was cleared. Pastor Tasha's son is currently performing at first grade level at 5 years old and refers to himself as Brilliant. Pastor Tasha Taylor was ordained as a Prophetess by Apostle Michael Hunter founder of Prophetic Minds Ministry in 2009 who also covered her newly established ministry, "Reaping Time Outreach Global." She was later covered by Apostle Anne Darville of Delray Beach.

Pastor Tasha was Ordained a Pastor by the covering Apostles Mitchells' of "DayStar Ministries."

Pastor Tasha Taylor started a ministry in Marietta, GA for prayer and Bible studies who meet in the Intown Suites Hotel located at: 2353 Barrett Creek Parkway, Marietta GA, 30066 on Sundays at 11am. She thrives on Prayer and generates the power to minister from the anointing. Her prayer services are privately held, but those who attend testify of the power of the Holy Ghost in her life, answers to prayer, and the move of the Spirit of God in their lives. She is also the author of five books: "Success that Begins When Asking for Help," "Marriage and Family," "Building Strong Families

in Critical Situations," "Human Development," and "Biblical Ethics: Finances."

Currently, "Reaping Time Outreach Worship Center" is covered under, The Apostolic Prophetic Connection with Ambassador Apostle Elizabeth Hairston McBurrows and Elder Carlton McBurrows.

Reaping Time Outreach Worship Center was Blessed and Pastor Tasha Taylor Ordained as Pastor on December 17, 2017 by Apostle Elizabeth Hairston McBurrows and Elder Carlton McBurrows. This ministry currently meets in a conference room at 6299 W. Sunrise Blvd. Plantation, FL Sundays 12 noon and Fridays at 5 pm and at 2300 Palm Beach Lakes Blvd. WPB, FL 33407, Sundays at 8 am and Tuesdays at 7 pm. To God be the Glory!!

"WORKS CITED"

[i] Romans 5:5

[ii] Heb. 6:4-6 It is impossible for those who have once been enlightened, who have tasted the heavenly gift, who have shared in the Holy Spirit, who have tasted the goodness of the word of God and the powers of the coming age— and then have fallen away—to be restored again to repentance, because they themselves are crucifying the Son of God all over again and subjecting Him to open shame....

[iii] ("Wikipedia") "Research has found that attempted suicide rates and suicidal ideation among lesbian, gay, bisexual, transgender, etc (LGBT) youth is significantly higher than among the general population.[1] LGBT youth have the highest rate of suicide attempts."

[iv] Mark 9:28-29 After Jesus had gone into the house, His disciples asked Him privately, "Why couldn't we drive it out?" 29Jesus answered, "This kind cannot come out, except by prayer."

[v] ("Bible Hub") power, authority, weight, especially: moral authority, influence, (b) in a quasi-personal sense, derived from later Judaism, of a spiritual power, and hence of an earthly power.

[vi] Matthew 10:32-33

[vii] Rom 14:11.

[viii]Luk. 1:7

[ix] Gen. 6:4.

[x] Gen. 6:8.

[xi] I Sam. 13:10.

[xii] II Sam. 11:12. 14 In the morning it happened that David wrote a letter to Joab and sent it by the hand of Uriah. 15 And he wrote in the letter, saying,

"Set Uriah in the forefront of the [c]hottest battle, and retreat from him, that he may be struck down and die." 16 So it was, while Joab besieged the city, that he assigned Uriah to a place where he knew there were valiant men. 17 Then the men of the city came out and fought with Joab. And some of the people of the servants of David fell; and Uriah the Hittite died also.

[xiii] Phi. 2:10.

[xiv] Isaiah 61.

[xv] Mat. 25:31-46.

[xvi] I Joh. 1:11-12.

[xvii] Hab. 2:4.

[xviii] Joh. 3:16.

xix Joh. 14:6-7. Jesus saith unto him, I am the way, the truth, and the life: no man cometh unto the Father, but by me. If ye had known me, ye should have known my Father also: and from henceforth ye know him, and have seen him.

xx Joh. 3:16.

xxi Pro. 31

xxii Deb. 4:9-23.

Made in the USA
Columbia, SC
28 January 2024

31060727R00058